Dr. Jane Frey

Breaking the Cycle of Chronic Back Pain

Diagnosis, Treatment and Prevention.

Contents

1

Introduction

Chronic back pain is a common medical condition that affects millions of people worldwide. It is defined as pain that persists for 12 weeks or longer, and it can have a significant impact on an individual's quality of life. Chronic back pain can be caused by a variety of factors, including injuries, degenerative diseases, and lifestyle factors. It can also be challenging to diagnose and treat, as the underlying causes can be complex and multi-factorial. This essay will explore the nature of chronic back pain, its impact on daily life, and the need for a comprehensive approach to managing this condition.

Understanding Chronic Back Pain

Chronic back pain is a complex medical condition that can be caused by a variety of factors. Injuries, such as those sustained in car accidents or sports activities, can lead to chronic back pain. Degenerative diseases, such as arthritis, spinal stenosis, and herniated discs, can also cause chronic back pain. Lifestyle factors, such as obesity, lack of exercise, and poor posture, can also contribute to chronic back pain. Psychological factors, such as stress and depression, can also play a role in the development and progression of chronic back pain.

The symptoms of chronic back pain can vary depending on the underlying cause. Common symptoms include a dull ache or sharp pain in the lower back, muscle stiffness, and difficulty moving. In some cases, chronic back pain can also lead to numbness, tingling, or weakness in the legs or feet. The severity of these symptoms can also vary, ranging from mild discomfort to debilitating pain that interferes with daily activities.

Diagnosing chronic back pain can be challenging, as the underlying causes can be complex and multi factorial. A comprehensive medical history and physical examination are typically the first steps in diagnosing chronic back pain. Imaging tests, such as X-rays, CT scans, and MRI scans, may also be used to help identify the underlying cause of chronic back pain. In some cases, blood tests and other diagnostic tests may also be necessary to help rule out underlying medical conditions that could be contributing to chronic back pain.

The Impact of Chronic Back Pain on Daily Life

Chronic back pain can have a significant impact on an individual's quality of life. It can interfere with daily activities, such as work, exercise, and social interactions. Chronic back pain can also lead to sleep disturbances, anxiety, and depression, which can further worsen the condition. The physical limitations caused by chronic back pain can also lead to a loss of independence and a decreased sense of self-worth.

The impact of chronic back pain can also extend beyond the individual to affect their family, friends, and caregivers. Family members and friends may need to provide support and assistance with daily activities, which can be stressful and time-consuming. Caregivers may also experience physical and emotional strain, leading to burnout and decreased quality of life.

The Need for a Comprehensive Approach to Managing Chronic Back Pain

Given the complex nature of chronic back pain, a comprehensive approach to managing this condition is necessary. A comprehensive approach should include a combination of medical, psychological, and lifestyle interventions to address the underlying causes and symptoms of chronic back pain.

Medical interventions for chronic back pain may include pain medications, physical therapy, and surgical interventions. Pain medications, such as non-steroidal anti-inflammatory drugs (NSAIDs), opioids, and muscle relaxants, can help alleviate pain and reduce inflammation. Physical therapy can help improve flexibility, strength, and posture, reducing the risk of further injury and improving overall function. Surgical interventions, such as spinal fusion or disk replacement surgery, may be necessary in severe cases of chronic back pain.

Psychological interventions for chronic back pain may include cognitive-behavioral therapy (CBT), mindfulness-based stress reduction (MBSR), and other forms of psychotherapy. CBT is a form of psychotherapy that focuses on identifying and changing negative thought patterns and behaviors that contribute to chronic back pain. CBT can help individuals with chronic back pain learn new coping skills, reduce stress and anxiety, and improve their overall quality of life. MBSR is another form of psychotherapy that uses mindfulness techniques, such as meditation and breathing exercises, to reduce stress and promote relaxation. MBSR has been shown to be effective in reducing chronic pain, including chronic back pain.

Lifestyle interventions for chronic back pain may include exercise, weight loss, and stress reduction techniques. Exercise, such as low-impact aerobic activity and strength training, can help improve flexibility, strength, and posture, reducing the risk of further injury and improving overall function. Weight loss can also help reduce the pressure on the spine, reducing pain and discomfort. Stress reduction techniques, such as yoga, meditation, and deep breathing, can help reduce stress and tension, promoting relaxation and reducing pain.

In addition to these interventions, a comprehensive approach to managing chronic back pain should also include patient education and support. Patient education can help individuals with chronic back pain understand their condition and develop a plan for managing their symptoms. Support from family, friends, and healthcare providers can also provide individuals with chronic back pain with the emotional and practical support they need to manage their condition effectively.

Chronic back pain is a complex medical condition that can have a significant impact on an individual's quality of life. The underlying causes of chronic back pain can be multi-factorial, making diagnosis and treatment challenging. A comprehensive approach to managing chronic back pain, including medical, psychological, and lifestyle interventions, is necessary to address the underlying causes and symptoms of this condition. Patient education and support are also essential components of effective chronic back pain management. By taking a comprehensive approach to managing chronic back pain, individuals with this condition can improve their quality of life and regain control over their health and well-being.

2

Causes of Chronic Back Pain

Chronic back pain is a common condition that affects millions of people worldwide. It is defined as pain in the back that lasts for more than three months. Chronic back pain can be caused by a variety of factors, and identifying the underlying cause is crucial to finding an effective treatment plan. In this article, we will discuss the different causes of chronic back pain, how to identify them, the mechanics of back pain, and the risk factors for developing chronic back pain.

Causes of Chronic Back Pain

There are numerous causes of chronic back pain. Some of the most common causes include:

1.Poor posture: Poor posture can put unnecessary strain on the back muscles and spine, leading to chronic back pain.

2.Herniated disc: A herniated disc occurs when the outer layer of a spinal disc ruptures, causing the gel-like material inside to leak out and press on the spinal nerves. This can cause chronic back pain.

3.Degenerative disc disease: As we age, the discs in our spine can degenerate and lose their cushioning ability. This can lead to chronic back pain.

4.Spinal stenosis: Spinal stenosis occurs when the spinal canal narrows, putting pressure on the spinal cord and nerves. This can cause chronic back pain.

5.Osteoarthritis: Osteoarthritis is a condition that causes the cartilage in our joints to break down, leading to pain and stiffness. This can also affect the joints in the back and cause chronic back pain.

6.Scoliosis: Scoliosis is a condition that causes the spine to curve sideways. This can cause chronic back pain, especially if the curve is severe.

7.Trauma: Trauma to the back, such as a car accident or fall, can cause chronic back pain.

8.Fibromyalgia: Fibromyalgia is a condition that causes widespread pain and tenderness throughout the body, including the back.

9.Obesity: Being overweight can put excess strain on the back muscles and spine, leading to chronic back pain.

Identifying the Different Causes of Chronic Back Pain

Identifying the underlying cause of chronic back pain is crucial to finding an effective treatment plan. Here are some of the ways doctors and healthcare providers can identify the different causes of chronic back pain:

1.Medical history: Doctors will typically start by taking a thorough medical history, including any previous injuries, surgeries, or conditions that could be contributing to the pain.

2.Physical examination: Doctors will typically perform a physical examination, checking for any signs of inflammation, muscle weakness, or limited range of motion.

3.Imaging tests: Imaging tests such as X-rays, CT scans, or MRI scans can help doctors identify any structural abnormalities in the spine, such as herniated discs or spinal stenosis.

4.Blood tests: Blood tests can help doctors rule out any underlying conditions, such as rheumatoid arthritis or infections, that could be causing the pain.

5.Nerve conduction studies: Nerve conduction studies can help doctors identify any nerve damage or dysfunction that could be causing the pain.

Understanding the Mechanics of Back Pain

To understand how chronic back pain occurs, it is important to understand the mechanics of the back. The back is made up of bones, muscles, ligaments, and nerves, all of which work together to provide support and mobility. When any of these structures are damaged or injured, it can lead to back pain. Here are some of the ways back pain can occur:

1.Muscle strain: Muscle strain occurs when the muscles in the back are stretched or torn, often due to poor posture or overuse.

2.Ligament sprain: Ligament sprains occur when the ligaments in the back are stretched or torn, often due to sudden twisting or turning movements, or from a traumatic injury such as a fall or collision.

Muscle strains and ligament sprains can both cause pain, swelling, and limited range of motion in the affected area. However, there are some key differences between the two conditions.

Muscle strains typically cause pain and discomfort when the muscle is actively used or stretched. The pain is often described as a dull ache or soreness, and may be accompanied by muscle spasms or stiffness.

Ligament sprains, on the other hand, typically cause pain and swelling around the affected joint, and may also cause instability or weakness in the joint. The pain is often described as sharp or shooting, and may be accompanied by a popping or tearing sensation at the time of injury.

Both muscle strains and ligament sprains can be treated with rest, ice, compression, and elevation (RICE) to reduce pain and swelling. Physical therapy and rehabilitation exercises may also be recommended to help restore strength, flexibility, and range of motion in the affected area. In more severe cases, surgery may be necessary to repair torn muscles or ligaments.

Risk factors for developing chronic back pain

Chronic back pain is a common condition that can significantly impact an individual's quality of life. It is defined as pain that persists for more than three months and can be caused by a variety of factors. Some of the risk factors for developing chronic back pain include:

*Age: As individuals age, the risk of developing chronic back pain increases. This is due to the natural wear and tear of the spine over time.

*Physical inactivity: A sedentary lifestyle can lead to weak muscles and poor posture, both of which can contribute to chronic back pain.

*Obesity: Being overweight or obese puts extra pressure on the spine and can increase the risk of developing chronic back pain.

*Poor posture: Poor posture, such as slouching or hunching over a desk, can put stress on the spine and lead to chronic back pain.

*Smoking: Smoking can cause damage to the discs in the spine and decrease blood flow, leading to chronic back pain.

*Stress: Chronic stress can lead to muscle tension and contribute to chronic back pain.

*Previous injury: A previous back injury can increase the risk of developing chronic back pain, especially if the injury was not properly treated or healed.

*Genetics: Certain genetic factors may predispose individuals to chronic back pain, such as inherited conditions that affect the spine.

*Occupational factors: Jobs that require heavy lifting, repetitive motions, or prolonged periods of sitting or standing can increase the risk of developing chronic back pain.

*Medical conditions: Certain medical conditions, such as arthritis or osteoporosis, can increase the risk of developing chronic back pain.

It is important to note that these risk factors do not necessarily guarantee the development of chronic back pain, but rather increase the likelihood. By taking steps to address these risk factors, such as maintaining a healthy weight, practicing good posture, and staying physically active, individuals can reduce their risk of developing chronic back pain.

3

Diagnosing Chronic Back Pain

Chronic back pain is a common condition that affects millions of people worldwide. It is defined as pain that persists for more than three months and is often associated with other symptoms such as stiffness, muscle spasms, and decreased mobility. The diagnosis of chronic back pain can be challenging, as there are many potential causes of the condition. In this article, we will discuss the diagnostic tools and tests used to diagnose chronic back pain, the role of imaging in the diagnosis process, and an understanding of the diagnostic process.

Diagnostic Tools and Tests for Chronic Back Pain

There are several diagnostic tools and tests used to diagnose chronic back pain. The first step in the diagnostic process is a thorough medical history and physical examination. The medical history should include questions about the duration, location, and severity of the pain, as well as any associated symptoms such as numbness, tingling, or weakness. The physical examination should include an assessment of range of motion, muscle strength, and reflexes.

Additional diagnostic tools that may be used to diagnose chronic back pain include blood tests, X-rays, CT scans, MRI scans, and nerve conduction studies.

Blood Tests

Blood tests are typically used to rule out underlying medical conditions that may be contributing to chronic back pain. For example, blood tests may be used to check for infections, autoimmune disorders, or cancer.

X-Rays

X-rays are commonly used to diagnose chronic back pain. They can help to identify structural abnormalities in the spine, such as herniated discs, fractures, or bone spurs. However, X-rays are not as useful for identifying soft tissue injuries, such as muscle strains or ligament sprains.

CT Scans

CT scans are similar to X-rays, but they provide more detailed images of the spine. CT scans are particularly useful for identifying fractures and other structural abnormalities that may be causing chronic back pain.

MRI Scans

MRI scans are often used to diagnose chronic back pain. They provide detailed images of the soft tissues in the spine, including the discs, nerves, and muscles. MRI scans are particularly useful for identifying herniated discs and other soft tissue injuries.

Nerve Conduction Studies

Nerve conduction studies are used to diagnose conditions that affect the nerves, such as sciatica or spinal stenosis. During the test, small electrical impulses are applied to the nerves in the affected area, and the response is measured. This can help to determine the extent of nerve damage and the underlying cause of chronic back pain.

The Role of Imaging in Diagnosing Chronic Back Pain

Imaging plays a crucial role in the diagnosis of chronic back pain. X-rays, CT scans, and MRI scans are the most commonly used imaging techniques.

1.X-rays: X-rays are often the first imaging test used to diagnose chronic back pain. They can provide a clear image of the bones in the spine, which can help to identify structural abnormalities such as fractures or bone spurs. X-rays are also useful for monitoring the progression of degenerative conditions, such as osteoarthritis.

2.CT Scans: CT scans are often used in conjunction with X-rays to provide more detailed images of the spine. They can help to identify fractures, herniated discs, and other structural abnormalities that may be causing chronic back pain.

3.MRI Scans: MRI scans are the most detailed imaging test used to diagnose chronic back pain. They can provide detailed images of the soft tissues in the spine, including the discs, nerves, and muscles. MRI scans are particularly useful for identifying herniated discs and other soft tissue injuries that may be contributing to chronic back pain.

Understanding the Diagnostic Process

The diagnostic process for chronic back pain can be complex, as there are many potential causes of the condition. However, there are several steps that are typically followed in the diagnostic process

Step 1: Medical

The first step in the diagnostic process for chronic back pain is a thorough medical history and physical examination. This involves gathering information about the patient's symptoms, including the duration, location, and severity of the pain, as well as any associated symptoms such as numbness, tingling, or weakness.

During the physical examination, the doctor will assess the patient's range of motion, muscle strength, and reflexes. They may also perform tests to identify areas of tenderness or pain in the back.

Based on the results of the medical history and physical examination, the doctor may order additional diagnostic tests to further evaluate the patient's condition.

Step 2: Diagnostic Tests

The second step in the diagnostic process for chronic back pain is to order diagnostic tests. These may include blood tests, X-rays, CT scans, MRI scans, and nerve conduction studies, as discussed earlier.

Blood tests may be ordered to rule out underlying medical conditions that may be contributing to chronic back pain. X-rays and CT scans can help to identify structural abnormalities in the spine, while MRI scans are particularly useful for identifying soft tissue injuries such as herniated discs.

Nerve conduction studies are used to diagnose conditions that affect the nerves, such as sciatica or spinal stenosis.

Step 3: Reviewing Results and Diagnosis

Once the diagnostic tests have been completed, the doctor will review the results to determine the underlying cause of the patient's chronic back pain.

Based on the results of the diagnostic tests, the doctor may make a diagnosis and recommend a course of treatment. Treatment options for chronic back pain may include medications, physical therapy, or surgery, depending on the underlying cause of the condition.

Step 4: Monitoring Progress

After treatment has been initiated, the doctor will monitor the patient's progress to determine if the treatment is effective. This may involve follow-up visits, additional diagnostic tests, and adjustments to the treatment plan as needed.

Diagnosing chronic back pain can be a complex and challenging process. A thorough medical history and physical examination are the first steps in the diagnostic process, followed by additional diagnostic tests such as blood tests, X-rays, CT scans, MRI scans, and nerve conduction studies.

Imaging plays a crucial role in the diagnosis of chronic back pain, providing detailed images of the spine that can help to identify structural abnormalities and soft tissue injuries.

Understanding the diagnostic process for chronic back pain is important for both patients and healthcare providers. By working together, patients and their doctors can develop an effective treatment plan to manage chronic back pain and improve quality of life.

4

Traditional Treatments for Chronic Back Pain

Chronic back pain is a common ailment that affects millions of people worldwide. It can be a debilitating condition that interferes with daily activities and reduces quality of life. Chronic back pain is defined as pain that lasts for more than 12 weeks and can be caused by a variety of factors such as injury, arthritis, or degenerative disc disease. While surgery is sometimes an option for chronic back pain, traditional treatments such as medications, physical therapy, and injections are often used first to manage the condition. In this essay, we will discuss these traditional treatments in detail.

Medications for Chronic Back Pain

Medications are a common treatment for chronic back pain,

and there are many different types available. The most commonly used medications for chronic back pain include:

1.Nonsteroidal anti-inflammatory drugs (NSAIDs): NSAIDs are a class of drugs that reduce inflammation and pain. They are available over-the-counter or by prescription and include drugs such as ibuprofen, naproxen, and aspirin. NSAIDs are typically the first-line treatment for chronic back pain and are effective in reducing pain and inflammation.

2.Acetaminophen: Acetaminophen is a pain reliever that is available over-the-counter. It is effective in reducing pain but does not reduce inflammation.

3.Muscle relaxants: Muscle relaxants are medications that help reduce muscle spasms and tightness. They are typically prescribed for short-term use because they can cause drowsiness and dizziness.

4.Opioids: Opioids are prescription pain medications that are effective in reducing pain. However, they are highly addictive and can cause side effects such as constipation, nausea, and dizziness. Opioids are typically prescribed for short-term use and only when other treatments have failed.

5.Antidepressants: Antidepressants are sometimes prescribed for chronic back pain because they can help reduce pain and improve mood. They are typically used in lower doses than when used to treat depression It is important to note that medications can have both benefits and risks, and should only be taken as directed by a healthcare professional. It's important to understand the potential benefits of a medication, as well as the potential risks and side effects. Some medications may be appropriate for certain individuals but not for others, and some may interact with other medications or medical conditions.

Additionally, it's important to follow the prescribed dosage and schedule of a medication, and to not stop taking it without consulting a healthcare professional. Abruptly stopping certain medications can lead to adverse effects, and may even be life-threatening in some cases.

Overall, medications can be a valuable tool in treating and managing various health conditions, but they should always be used with caution and under the guidance of a healthcare professional.

Physical therapy for chronic back Pain

Physical therapy is a non-invasive and effective treatment option for managing chronic back pain.

Physical therapy for chronic back pain typically involves a combination of exercises, stretches, and manual therapies. The goals of physical therapy are to reduce pain, improve mobility and flexibility, and strengthen the muscles of the back and core.

One common exercise used in physical therapy for chronic back pain is the McKenzie Method. This method involves a series of movements and positions that can help relieve pressure on the spine and reduce pain. Another exercise commonly used in physical therapy is the lumbar stabilization exercise, which aims to strengthen the muscles of the lower back and improve posture.

Manual therapies, such as massage and spinal manipulation, may also be used in physical therapy for chronic back pain. These techniques can help improve blood flow to the affected area, reduce inflammation, and improve range of motion.

Physical therapy for chronic back pain may also involve education on proper body mechanics and posture, as well as tips for preventing future back pain. This can include strategies such as proper lifting techniques and ergonomics in the workplace.

Overall, physical therapy is a safe and effective treatment

option for managing chronic back pain. It can help reduce pain, improve mobility and flexibility, and strengthen the muscles of the back and core, leading to improved overall quality of life. If you are experiencing chronic back pain, consult with a healthcare professional to determine if physical therapy may be right for you.

Injections for chronic back pain

It is a debilitating condition that can have a significant impact on an individual's quality of life. Injections are one of the treatment options available for chronic back pain. In this article, we will discuss the different types of injections used to treat chronic back pain.

1.Epidural steroid injections (ESIs) Epidural steroid injections (ESIs) are one of the most commonly used injections for chronic back pain. They are used to reduce inflammation and relieve pain in the spinal area. ESIs involve injecting a mixture of steroids and a local anesthetic directly into the epidural space of the spine. The epidural space is the area that surrounds the spinal cord and the nerves that branch off from it. ESIs are usually performed under fluoroscopy or X-ray guidance to ensure accurate placement of the needle.

2.Facet joint injections Facet joints are small joints located between each vertebra in the spine. They provide stability and allow for movement in the spine. Facet joint injections involve injecting a mixture of local anesthetic and steroid medication directly into the facet joint. This injection can provide relief from pain caused by inflammation or irritation of the facet joint.

3.Sacroiliac joint injections The sacroiliac joint is located in the lower back and connects the sacrum to the pelvis. It is a common site of pain in individuals with chronic back pain. Sacroiliac joint injections involve injecting a mixture of local anesthetic and steroid medication directly into the joint. This injection can provide relief from pain caused by inflammation or irritation of the sacroiliac joint.

4.Trigger point injections Trigger points are areas of muscle that are tender to the touch and can cause pain. Trigger point injections involve injecting a local anesthetic directly into the trigger point to provide relief from pain.

Injections for chronic back pain are usually performed as an outpatient procedure and can provide long-lasting relief from pain. However, injections are not suitable for everyone, and their effectiveness varies from person to person. It is essential to discuss the benefits and risks of injections with your healthcare provider to determine if they are the right treatment option for you.

5

Alternative Treatments for Chronic Back Pain

It is a complex condition that is often challenging to treat using conventional therapies such as medication and surgery. Alternative therapies such as acupuncture, chiropractic care, and massage therapy have been gaining popularity as effective treatments for chronic back pain. This book aims to provide an overview of these alternative therapies and their effectiveness in treating chronic back pain.

Acupuncture for Chronic Back Pain

Acupuncture is a traditional Chinese medicine therapy that involves the insertion of thin needles into specific points on the body. The practice is based on the concept that the human body has energy channels known as meridians, and the stimulation of specific points on these meridians can help restore the balance of energy flow in the body.

Acupuncture has been shown to be effective in treating chronic back pain. A systematic review and meta-analysis of 29 randomized controlled trials (RCTs) involving 17,922 patients found that acupuncture was more effective than sham acupuncture, no acupuncture, or conventional therapies for the treatment of chronic back pain (Vickers et al., 2012). The study also found that the effect of acupuncture was long-lasting and that the benefits were evident even after six months of treatment.

Another study published in the Annals of Internal Medicine compared the effectiveness of acupuncture and usual care for the treatment of chronic back pain in 638 patients. The study found that acupuncture was significantly more effective than usual care in reducing back pain intensity and improving functional status (Cherkin et al., 2009).

The mechanism of action of acupuncture in treating chronic back pain is not entirely understood. However, it is believed that the insertion of needles stimulates the release of endorphins, which are natural painkillers produced by the body. Acupuncture may also reduce inflammation and promote healing by increasing blood flow to the affected area.

Chiropractic Care for Chronic Back Pain

Chiropractic care is a complementary therapy that involves the manipulation of the spine and other joints to alleviate pain and improve function. Chiropractic care is based on the principle that misalignments of the spine (subluxations) can interfere with the nervous system's proper functioning, leading to pain and other health problems.

Several studies have shown that chiropractic care is effective in treating chronic back pain. A systematic review and meta-analysis of 26 RCTs involving 1,743 patients found that spinal manipulation was more effective than sham manipulation, no treatment, or other therapies for the treatment of chronic low back pain (Rubinstein et al., 2011). The study also found that the benefits of chiropractic care were evident even after 12 months of treatment.

Another study published in the Journal of Manipulative and Physiological Therapeutics compared the effectiveness of chiropractic care and medical care for the treatment of chronic low back pain in 278 patients. The study found that chiropractic care was more effective than medical care in reducing pain and improving function (Nyiendo et al., 2000).

The mechanism of action of chiropractic care in treating

chronic back pain is not entirely understood. However, it is believed that spinal manipulation may reduce pain by restoring normal joint motion, reducing inflammation, and improving nerve function.

Massage Therapy for Chronic Back Pain

Massage therapy is a manual therapy that involves the manipulation of soft tissues such as muscles, tendons, and ligaments to alleviate pain and improve function. Massage therapy can be performed using different techniques, such as Swedish massage, deep tissue massage, and trigger point therapy.

Several studies have shown that massage therapy is effective in treating chronic back pain. A systematic review and meta-analysis of 25 RCTs involving 3,096 patients found that massage therapy was more effective than no treatment, sham treatment, or other therapies for the treatment of chronic back pain (Cherkin et al., 2011). The study found that the benefits of massage therapy were evident even after six months of treatment.

Another study published in the Annals of Internal Medicine compared the effectiveness of massage therapy and usual care for the treatment of chronic low back pain in 401 patients. The study found that massage therapy was more effective than usual care in reducing pain and improving function (Cherkin et al., 2011).

The mechanism of action of massage therapy in treating chronic back pain is not entirely understood. However, it is believed that massage therapy may reduce pain by increasing blood flow to the affected area, reducing muscle tension, and promoting relaxation.

Chronic back pain is a prevalent health problem that can significantly affect a person's quality of life. Alternative therapies such as acupuncture, chiropractic care, and massage therapy have been gaining popularity as effective treatments for chronic back pain. These therapies have been shown to be more effective than conventional therapies such as medication and surgery and have fewer side effects. However, it is essential to note that these therapies may not be suitable for everyone, and patients should consult with their healthcare provider before trying any alternative therapy.

Further research is needed to understand the mechanisms of action of these therapies better and to determine which patients are most likely to benefit from them. Despite the need for more research, alternative therapies such as acupuncture, chiropractic care, and massage therapy offer promising options for the treatment of chronic back pain and may help improve the quality of life for millions of people worldwide.

6

Lifestyle Changes to Prevent Chronic Back Pain

Chronic back pain can be debilitating and can significantly impact an individual's quality of life. It is important to take proactive steps to prevent back pain, as opposed to waiting for it to occur and then seeking treatment. Lifestyle changes such as exercise, maintaining good posture, and proper nutrition can help prevent chronic back pain. In this article, we will discuss the importance of exercise, maintaining good posture, and proper nutrition for preventing chronic back pain.

The importance of exercise for preventing chronic back pain

Regular exercise is one of the most effective ways to prevent chronic back pain. Exercise helps strengthen the muscles that support the spine, which can reduce the risk of injury and strain. It also helps maintain flexibility and range of motion, which can reduce stiffness and pain.

There are many types of exercises that can be beneficial for preventing chronic back pain. Low-impact aerobic exercises, such as walking, cycling, and swimming, can help improve cardiovascular health and increase endurance. These types of exercises are also gentle on the joints and can help improve flexibility.

Strength training exercises, such as weight lifting and resistance training, can help build muscle and improve posture. Strong muscles can help support the spine and reduce the risk of injury. Yoga and Pilates are also effective exercises for preventing chronic back pain, as they focus on improving flexibility, strength, and balance.

It is important to consult with a healthcare provider before beginning any exercise program. A healthcare provider can recommend the best type of exercise for an individual's specific needs and medical conditions.

Maintaining good posture to prevent chronic back pain

Maintaining good posture is essential for preventing chronic back pain. Poor posture can put undue stress on the spine, which can lead to pain and injury over time. Good posture involves sitting and standing with the spine in a neutral position, which means that the natural curves of the spine are maintained.

When sitting, it is important to sit with the back straight and the feet flat on the floor. The hips should be positioned at the back of the chair, and the shoulders should be relaxed. The computer screen should be at eye level, and the keyboard should be at a comfortable height.

When standing, it is important to stand with the shoulders back and the hips aligned with the ankles. The weight should be evenly distributed on both feet, and the knees should be slightly bent. High-heeled shoes should be avoided, as they can alter the alignment of the spine and cause back pain.

It is important to take frequent breaks when sitting for long periods of time. Standing up and stretching can help relieve tension and reduce the risk of injury. It is also important to avoid slouching or hunching over, as this can put undue stress on the spine.

Nutrition and chronic back pain prevention

Proper nutrition is important for overall health and can also help prevent chronic back pain. Eating a balanced diet that includes fruits, vegetables, whole grains, lean protein, and healthy fats can help reduce inflammation, improve circulation, and promote healing.

Inflammation is a common cause of chronic back pain. Certain foods can increase inflammation in the body, while others can help reduce it. Foods that can increase inflammation include processed foods, sugar, and saturated fats. Foods that can help reduce inflammation include omega-3 fatty acids, which are found in fish, nuts, and seeds, and antioxidants, which are found in fruits and vegetables.

Calcium and vitamin D are essential nutrients for bone health. Strong bones can help support the spine and reduce the risk of injury. Foods that are high in calcium include dairy products, leafy green vegetables, and fortified foods. Vitamin D is found in fatty fish, egg yolks, and fortified foods. It is also produced by the body when the skin is exposed to sunlight. Supplements may be necessary for individuals who are not able to get enough calcium and vitamin D from their diet or exposure to sunlight. It is important to talk to a healthcare provider before starting any supplements, as excessive amounts can be harmful.

Dehydration can also contribute to chronic back pain. Staying hydrated can help keep the intervertebral discs in the spine hydrated and healthy. It is recommended to drink at least 8 cups of water per day, and more during periods of increased activity or hot weather.

In addition to proper nutrition, maintaining a healthy weight is important for preventing chronic back pain. Excess weight can put undue stress on the spine and increase the risk of injury. Losing weight can help reduce the risk of chronic back pain and improve overall health.

Chronic back pain can significantly impact an individual's quality of life. Fortunately, there are steps that can be taken to prevent chronic back pain. Regular exercise, maintaining good posture, and proper nutrition are all important for preventing chronic back pain. It is important to consult with a healthcare provider before starting any exercise program or supplements, as they can recommend the best course of action for an individual's specific needs and medical conditions. By taking proactive steps to prevent chronic back pain, individuals can improve their overall health and well-being.

7

Coping with Chronic Back Pain

The prevalence of chronic back pain has been on the rise, and it is one of the leading causes of disability and work absenteeism. The condition is multifactorial and can be caused by various factors, including injury, poor posture, obesity, and psychological factors such as stress, anxiety, and depression. Chronic back pain can be debilitating, affecting a person's quality of life, and managing it can be challenging. This article explores various psychological approaches and mind–body practices that can help manage chronic back pain. Additionally, the article looks at the role of support groups in the management of chronic back pain.

Psychological Approaches to Managing Chronic Back Pain

Chronic back pain has both physical and psychological

components. Psychological factors, such as stress, anxiety, depression, and fear, can exacerbate the pain experience, leading to reduced functioning and poor quality of life. Psychological interventions, such as cognitive-behavioral therapy (CBT), mindfulness-based stress reduction (MBSR), and acceptance and commitment therapy (ACT), have been shown to be effective in managing chronic back pain.

Cognitive-behavioral therapy (CBT) is a psychological intervention that focuses on changing negative thought patterns and behaviors that may be contributing to the pain experience. CBT aims to help individuals identify and challenge negative thoughts and replace them with more positive and realistic ones. It also helps individuals develop coping skills to manage the pain and improve functioning. Several studies have shown that CBT can reduce pain intensity, improve physical function, and reduce disability in individuals with chronic back pain.

Mindfulness-based stress reduction (MBSR) is another psychological intervention that has been shown to be effective in managing chronic back pain. MBSR combines mindfulness meditation, yoga, and body awareness techniques to help individuals manage stress and improve pain coping skills. MBSR has been shown to reduce pain intensity, improve mood, and improve quality of life in individuals with chronic back pain.

Acceptance and commitment therapy (ACT) is a psychological intervention that aims to help individuals accept their pain experience while committing to actions that align with their values. ACT involves mindfulness-based techniques, such as acceptance and cognitive defusion, to help individuals manage the emotional distress associated with chronic pain. Studies have shown that ACT can improve pain acceptance, reduce pain-related anxiety, and improve functioning in individuals with chronic back pain.

Mind-Body Practices for Managing Chronic Back Pain

Mind-body practices refer to techniques that combine physical and mental activities to promote overall health and wellbeing. These practices include yoga, tai chi, meditation, and deep breathing exercises. Mind-body practices have been shown to be effective in managing chronic back pain by reducing pain intensity, improving physical function, and reducing emotional distress.

Yoga is a mind-body practice that combines physical postures, breathing exercises, and meditation to promote relaxation and reduce stress. Yoga has been shown to reduce pain intensity, improve physical function, and improve quality of life in individuals with chronic back pain. The physical postures in yoga help to improve flexibility, strength, and posture, which can alleviate back pain. Breathing exercises and meditation in yoga help to reduce stress and improve pain coping skills.

Tai chi is another mind-body practice that has been shown to be effective in managing chronic back pain. Tai chi involves slow and gentle movements that are coordinated with deep breathing and meditation. Tai chi has been shown to reduce pain intensity, improve physical function, and reduce emotional distress in individuals with chronic back pain. The slow and gentle movements in tai chi help to improve balance, flexibility, and posture, which can alleviate back pain.

In addition to yoga and tai chi, meditation and deep breathing exercises have also been shown to be effective in managing chronic back pain. Meditation involves focusing the mind on a specific object, thought, or activity to promote relaxation and reduce stress. Deep breathing exercises involve slow and deep breaths that help to calm the mind and reduce muscle tension.

Studies have shown that mindfulness meditation can reduce pain intensity, improve physical function, and reduce emotional distress in individuals with chronic back pain. Deep breathing exercises, such as diaphragmatic breathing and paced respiration, have also been shown to reduce pain intensity and improve physical function in individuals with chronic back pain.

Support Groups for Chronic Back Pain

Support groups are groups of individuals who share a common experience or condition and come together to provide emotional and social support to one another. Support groups for chronic back pain provide a safe and supportive environment for individuals to share their experiences, feelings, and coping strategies. These groups can also provide practical advice and resources for managing chronic back pain.

Research has shown that support groups for chronic pain can reduce pain intensity, improve mood, and improve quality of life in individuals with chronic pain (8). Support groups can also help to reduce feelings of isolation and promote social connectedness, which can improve emotional wellbeing.

In addition to in-person support groups, online support groups have also become increasingly popular. Online support groups provide individuals with a convenient and accessible way to connect with others who are experiencing similar challenges. Online support groups can also provide anonymity, which can be particularly beneficial for individuals who may feel uncomfortable sharing their experiences in person.

Chronic back pain is a complex and challenging condition that can have physical, emotional, and social impacts. Psychological approaches, such as cognitive-behavioral therapy, mindfulness-based stress reduction, and acceptance and commitment therapy, have been shown to be effective in managing chronic back pain. Mind-body practices, such as yoga, tai chi, meditation, and deep breathing exercises, can also be effective in reducing pain intensity, improving physical function, and reducing emotional distress. Support groups, both in-person and online, can provide emotional and social support, as well as practical advice and resources, for individuals with chronic back pain. It is important for individuals with chronic back pain to work with their healthcare providers to develop a comprehensive treatment plan that addresses all aspects of the condition.

8

Prevention Strategies for Chronic Back Pain

Chronic back pain can have a significant impact on an individual's quality of life, causing them to miss work, social activities, and even daily tasks. Fortunately, there are many strategies that individuals can employ to prevent chronic back pain. In this essay, we will discuss prevention strategies for chronic back pain, including ergonomic workplace practices, preventing sports-related back injuries, and preventing back pain while lifting heavy objects.

Ergonomic Workplace Practices to Prevent Chronic Back Pain

The workplace is a common place where people experience back pain. Most individuals spend a significant amount of time sitting at a desk, which can lead to poor posture and back pain. Ergonomic workplace practices can help prevent chronic back pain by reducing the strain on the back and promoting good posture.

One of the most important ergonomic practices to prevent back pain is to have a properly designed workstation. This includes having an adjustable chair, keyboard, and monitor. The chair should be adjustable to ensure that the individual's feet are flat on the floor, and the knees are at a 90-degree angle. The keyboard should be positioned so that the elbows are at a 90-degree angle, and the monitor should be at eye level to reduce neck strain.

Another important ergonomic practice to prevent back pain is to take frequent breaks. Sitting for long periods of time can put a lot of pressure on the back, leading to chronic pain. Taking a break every 30 minutes to stretch or walk around can help alleviate this pressure and reduce the risk of chronic back pain.

In addition to having a properly designed workstation and taking frequent breaks, individuals can also use ergonomic accessories to prevent back pain. For example, using a lumbar support pillow can help maintain proper posture and reduce the strain on the lower back. Similarly, using a footrest can help maintain proper alignment of the spine.

Preventing Sports-Related Back Injuries

Sports-related back injuries are a common cause of chronic back pain. Athletes who participate in contact sports, such as football or rugby, are at a higher risk of experiencing back injuries. However, individuals who participate in non-contact sports, such as running or tennis, can also experience back injuries.

One of the most important strategies to prevent sports-related back injuries is to warm up properly before participating in any physical activity. Warming up can help prepare the muscles and joints for the activity, reducing the risk of injury. A proper warm-up should include stretching, light cardio, and dynamic movements.

Another important strategy to prevent sports-related back injuries is to use proper technique. Athletes should be trained on the proper technique for their specific sport and should be encouraged to use proper technique during every practice and game. Using improper technique can put unnecessary strain on the back, leading to chronic pain and injury.

In addition to warming up properly and using proper technique, athletes should also wear proper gear. For contact sports, this may include wearing protective equipment such as helmets and padding. For non-contact sports, this may include wearing appropriate shoes and clothing.

Preventing Back Pain While Lifting Heavy Objects

Lifting heavy objects is a common cause of back pain. Whether it's lifting weights at the gym or lifting boxes at work, improper lifting techniques can lead to chronic back pain. Fortunately, there are many strategies that individuals can employ to prevent back pain while lifting heavy objects.

One of the most important strategies to prevent back pain while lifting heavy objects is to use proper lifting technique. The proper technique involves bending at the knees and keeping the back straight while lifting. It is also important to lift with the legs rather than the back. This technique helps to distribute the weight evenly and reduces the strain on the back.

Another important strategy to prevent back pain while lifting heavy objects is to use proper lifting equipment. This may include using a lifting belts, gloves, or straps to help support the back and reduce the risk of injury. Lifting belts, in particular, can provide extra support to the lower back muscles and reduce the pressure on the spine during heavy lifting.

It is also important to avoid lifting objects that are too heavy or awkward to lift alone. If an object is too heavy, individuals should ask for help or use equipment, such as a dolly or forklift, to move the object safely. Similarly, if an object is too awkward to lift alone, individuals should use teamwork or lifting aids to safely move the object.

Proper planning and organization can also help prevent back pain while lifting heavy objects. Individuals should plan their lift, including identifying the weight and size of the object, the lifting technique to use, and the proper lifting equipment. By planning ahead, individuals can reduce the risk of injury and ensure that the lift is performed safely.

Chronic back pain is a common health condition that can have a significant impact on an individual's quality of life. Fortunately, there are many strategies that individuals can employ to prevent chronic back pain. Ergonomic workplace practices, preventing sports-related back injuries, and preventing back pain while lifting heavy objects are all effective strategies for preventing chronic back pain. By incorporating these strategies into daily routines, individuals can reduce the risk of chronic back pain and maintain good spinal health.

9

Conclusion

Chronic back pain is a complex and debilitating condition that affects millions of people worldwide. It can significantly impact an individual's quality of life, limiting their ability to perform daily tasks and even leading to depression and anxiety. Despite the prevalence of chronic back pain, there is no one-size-fits-all solution for managing it. Instead, a comprehensive approach that includes various strategies is necessary to break the cycle of chronic back pain and improve an individual's overall health and well-being.

This book has explored the different aspects of managing chronic back pain. It has discussed the importance of seeking medical advice to rule out any underlying conditions, such as spinal stenosis or herniated discs. It has also highlighted the role of physical therapy, exercise, and proper posture in managing chronic back pain. In addition, this essay has discussed the potential benefits of alternative therapies, such as acupuncture and massage, in managing chronic back pain.

Perhaps the most crucial aspect of managing chronic back pain is taking an active role in your own care. This means empowering yourself to break the cycle of chronic pain through self-care and lifestyle changes. It requires making changes to your diet, sleeping habits, and stress management techniques. It also requires adopting a positive mindset and seeking support from friends, family, and healthcare professionals.

By taking an active role in your care, you can reduce the severity and frequency of chronic back pain episodes. You can also improve your overall health and well-being, allowing you to live a more fulfilling life. It is essential to remember that managing chronic back pain is a process that requires patience and perseverance. However, by adopting a comprehensive approach and empowering yourself to break the cycle of chronic pain, you can take control of your health and live a happier, healthier life.

Empowering Yourself to Break the Cycle of Chronic Back Pain

As discussed earlier, chronic back pain can significantly

impact an individual's quality of life. It can limit their ability to perform daily tasks, affect their mood, and even lead to depression and anxiety. Unfortunately, many people who suffer from chronic back pain rely solely on medication to manage their symptoms. While medication can be helpful in some cases, it is not a long-term solution.

To break the cycle of chronic back pain, it is essential to empower yourself and take an active role in your care. This requires making lifestyle changes and adopting self-care strategies that can help reduce the severity and frequency of chronic pain episodes.

1.Exercise and Physical Therapy

One of the most effective ways to manage chronic back pain is through exercise and physical therapy. Exercise can help strengthen the muscles in your back, reducing the strain on your spine and improving your overall posture. Physical therapy can also help improve your range of motion and flexibility, reducing the risk of future injuries.

It is essential to work with a qualified physical therapist who can create a personalized exercise program that meets your needs. This can include exercises that target specific muscles in your back, as well as stretches that help improve your range of motion. By incorporating exercise and physical therapy into your routine, you can reduce the severity and frequency of chronic pain episodes and improve your overall health and well-being.

2.Alternative Therapies

In addition to exercise and physical therapy, alternative therapies such as acupuncture and massage can also be helpful in managing chronic back pain. Acupuncture involves the insertion of fine needles into specific points on the body to promote healing and reduce pain. Massage can help relax the muscles in your back, improving circulation and reducing tension.

While alternative therapies may not work for everyone, they can be helpful for some individuals. It is essential to work with a qualified practitioner who has experience treating chronic back pain. By incorporating alternative therapies into your care plan, you can reduce the severity and frequency of chronic pain episodes and improve your overall well-being

3.Diet and Nutrition

Diet and nutrition play a crucial role in managing chronic back pain. Eating a healthy diet can help reduce inflammation in the body, which can contribute to chronic pain. It can also help you maintain a healthy weight, reducing the strain on your back muscles and spine.

It is essential to work with a registered dietitian who can create a personalized nutrition plan that meets your needs. This may include incorporating more anti-inflammatory foods into your diet, such as leafy greens, berries, and fatty fish. It may also involve reducing your intake of processed and sugary foods, which can contribute to inflammation and weight gain. By making dietary changes, you can improve your overall health and reduce the severity and frequency of chronic pain episodes.

4.Sleep

Getting enough sleep is essential for managing chronic back pain. Lack of sleep can increase inflammation in the body, contributing to chronic pain. It can also increase stress levels, making it more difficult to manage pain.

To improve your sleep quality, it is essential to create a relaxing bedtime routine. This may include avoiding electronic devices before bedtime, practicing relaxation techniques such as deep breathing or meditation, and ensuring your sleeping environment is comfortable and conducive to sleep. By improving your sleep quality, you can reduce the severity and frequency of chronic pain episodes and improve your overall health and well-being.

5.Stress Management

Stress can contribute to chronic back pain by increasing tension in the muscles and increasing inflammation in the body. Therefore, stress management techniques such as meditation, yoga, and deep breathing can be helpful in managing chronic back pain.

It is essential to find stress management techniques that work for you and incorporate them into your daily routine. This may involve taking a few minutes each day to practice deep breathing or incorporating yoga or meditation into your exercise routine. By managing stress, you can reduce the severity and frequency of chronic pain episodes and improve your overall health and well-being.

6.Positive Mindset

Finally, it is essential to maintain a positive mindset when managing chronic back pain. Chronic pain can be challenging to manage, and it is easy to become discouraged or frustrated. However, adopting a positive attitude can help you stay motivated and focused on your goals.

It is essential to find activities or hobbies that bring you joy and focus on the things you can do, rather than the things you cannot do. This may involve finding new hobbies that are less physically demanding or focusing on activities that do not aggravate your pain. By maintaining a positive attitude, you can reduce stress and improve your overall health and well-being.

Chronic back pain is a complex and debilitating condition that can significantly impact an individual's quality of life. While medication may provide temporary relief, a comprehensive approach that includes various strategies is necessary to break the cycle of chronic pain and improve an individual's overall health and well-being. Empowering yourself to take an active role in your care, through self-care and lifestyle changes, can help reduce the severity and frequency of chronic pain episodes and improve your overall health and well-being. It is essential to work with qualified healthcare professionals and find strategies that work for you to manage chronic back pain effectively. By adopting a comprehensive approach and empowering yourself to take control of your health, you can live a happier, healthier life.